FLAT BELLY: START LOSING WEIGHT RIGHT NOW!

Full 14 Day Flat Belly Healthy Eating Meal Plan!

POCKET GUIDE TO

A FLAT BELLY DIET AND FLAT BELLY RECIPES FOR EVERYONE

INTRODUCTION

Want to start eating healthier and lose weight now? These simple and tasty recipes that make up our Full 14 Day Flat Belly Healthy Eating Meal Plan, will help make the journey easy and delicious! You can try out the full plan or simply take some of your favourite recipes and incorporate them into the diet you have now. Enjoy!

Starting Notes:

1. Best Ingredients Possible: pick organic and/or grass fed options whenever possible.

2. Pass On The Processed. You'll notice this plan eliminates processed foods; aim to avoid processed foods whenever possible. When you do need processed options, look for choices with recognizable, whole food ingredients.

3. Be Flexible. If you see an ingredient you don't care for or are allergic to, simply replace it with a like ingredient. For example, if you can't have shrimp, just replace it with another lean protein and you'll be all set!

4. Drink Water! Aim for 2 litres a day.

Be sure to consult with a medical professional before changing your diet or fitness regime!

Full 14 Day Flat Belly Healthy Eating Meal Plan!

Healthy Eating Meal Plan – Day 1

Breakfast:
Veggie Packed Frittata.
Frittatas are a perfect way to start your day with veggies and protein. Another plus about frittatas? They're a perfect option to make ahead and heat up quickly in the morning.

Veggie Frittata:
What You'll Need:
1 tbs. butter or margarine
1 cup sliced mushrooms
1/2 cup chopped green and/or red peppers
1/3 cup chopped onion
12 eggs
1/4 cup water

How to Make It:
Melt butter in a medium (10-inch/25 cm) frying pan over medium heat. Add mushrooms, peppers and onion; saute until tender.
While vegetables are cooking, whisk together eggs and water. Pour egg mixture over vegetables in the frying pan. Cover and cook over medium heat, occasionally poking through the mixture to allow uncooked egg to flow to the bottom of the pan.
When bottom is cooked and top is almost set, finish cooking the frittata on the stove top by covering it with a lid for a few minutes, or flip it over in the pan to cook the top, or cook the top under the broiler.
To flip the frittata, place a dinner plate over the pan holding it firmly in place, then turn the frying pan and plate upside down. The frittata will fall into the plate, top side down. Slide the frittata back into the frying pan, top down. Cook for a few minutes until top (now the bottom) is cooked.

Alternately, place the frying pan under a preheated broiler until the top is cooked and slightly puffed, about a minute or two. The frying pan must be ovenproof in order to do this. To ovenproof the handle, wrap it with a double thickness of aluminum foil.
Cut into wedges and serve.

Lunch:
Easy Burritos.
Making a simple burrito is a great way to have a simple healthy lunch filled with protein and fiber. All you need to do is fill a whole grain tortilla with beans, spinach leafs, and a small amount of cheese and heat in the microwave. Garnish with as much salsa as you like, but be sure to check that your salsa choice has no added sugars.

Dinner:
Southwestern Stuffed Spaghetti Squash.
Spaghetti squash is a great, antioxidant packed alternative to the refined carbs found in most conventional pastas. Prepare this healthy and tasty stuffed spaghetti squash for a complete meal in one dish.

What You'll Need:
1 spaghetti squash
2 tbs. extra-virgin olive oil
1/2 red onion, chopped
3 garlic cloves, minced
1 jalapeno pepper, minced (leave seeds in for more heat)
1 red bell pepper, chopped
1 tbs. ground cumin
1 tbs. Mexican oregano
1 tbs. chili powder
1 can black beans (drained and rinsed)
1 cup frozen corn, thawed
coarse salt and freshly ground pepper
1/2 cup freshly torn cilantro, plus more for garnish
1 lime1 cup grated cheddar cheese

How to Make It:

Preheat oven to 375 F.

Roast squash on a baking sheet for 50 minutes. Let cool another 30 minutes, then cut in half. Spoon out the seeds, then using a fork, scrape up the flesh, making the "spaghetti."

Heat oil in a medium skillet. Add the onion, garlic, jalapeno pepper and red bell pepper. Saute 2 minutes. Add cumin, Mexican oregano, chili powder and a good pinch of salt and pepper. Saute another minute. Add the beans, corn and cilantro. Stir to combine. Squeeze in the lime juice and give one last stir.

Add in half the "spaghetti" to the bean mixture and stir to combine. Taste and season accordingly. I probably tossed in a little more salt at this point.

Switch oven to broil.

Stuff each squash half with the mixture and top with grated cheese.

Stick it back under the broiler until the cheese melts and gets all brown and bubbly.

Garnish with a leetle bit of cilantro and enjoy your life.

Snack:

Faux Cream.

Want all the goodness of ice cream in a dish that's actually good for you? Freeze one banana and combine it with a tablespoon of your favorite nut butter in the blender for a faux ice cream that you'll love.

Healthy Eating Meal Plan – Day 2

Breakfast:
Overnight Oats.
A hearty healthy breakfast packed with fiber, vitamins, and nutrients... in a jar (no cooking required)!

What You'll Need:
1/4 cup quick oats
1/2 cup unsweetened almond milk (or skim, soy)
1/4 medium banana, sliced (freeze the rest for smoothies!)
1/2 tbs. chia seeds
1/2 cup blueberries
4-5 drops liquid vanilla stevia (or your favorite sweetener)
pinch cinnamon
for the topping:
1 tbs chopped pecans (or any nut)

How to Make It:
Place all the ingredient in a jar, shake, cover and refrigerate overnight. Add your favorite crunchy toppings such as nuts, granola and enjoy the next day!

Lunch:
Lettuce Wraps.
Skip the carb loaded bread and effortlessly add extra greens to your lunch by skipping the bread on your favorite sandwich in favor of wrapping up your sandwich in large lettuce leaves.

Dinner:
Salmon and asparagus.
Salmon is loaded with healthy benefits for your heart and brain. Aim to have it once a week.

What You'll Need:
1 large salmon filet
1 bag of frozen brussel sprouts
1 bunch of thin asparagus

2 tbs. of olive oil
2 tbs. of butter
Garlic salt, salt and pepper, fish seasoning

How to Make It:
Place the salmon skin side down in the middle of the pan.
Trick for cooking brussel sprouts is to buy them frozen the in ready to steam bag. Cook them as directed on the package. Once they are cooked put them on one side of the salmon. Place the raw asparagus on the other side of the of the salmon.
Drizzle olive oil over both vegetables and sprinkle with garlic salt.
Sprinkle your salmon with salt, pepper, garlic salt, and fish seasoning.
Cut your butter into small chunks and place it all on top of your salmon.
Bake at 400 F for 20 minutes (or until salmon is cooked through - check the thickest spot)

Snack:
Fruit and Veggie Chips.
Thinly slice apples, bananas, and sweet potatoes and bake at 200 F until crispy.

Healthy Eating Meal Plan – Day 3

Breakfast:
Super Toast.
Top a piece of whole grain toast with thinly sliced avocado and an egg cooked however you prefer. This satisfying breakfast has everything you need to keep you going all morning.

Lunch:
A Better PBJ.
Ditch the sugary kids version of a peanut butter and jelly in favor of this tasty grown up alternative. Spread your favorite peanut butter or nut butter (check to make sure it has no added sugars!) on a low carb tortilla and top with finely chopped berries. Enjoy a side of kale chips.

Dinner:
Turkey Burgers.
Looking to mix it up from traditional burgers? Try these tasty and healthy turkey burgers. Use thick slices of tomato or large leaves of lettuce in lieu of bun. Top with leftover avocado from breakfast and serve with a side of oven baked sweet potato fries.

What You'll Need:
1 16- to 20-inch-long baguette, preferably whole-grain
1 large red onion, cut into 1/4-inch-thick rounds, divided
1 pound 93%-lean ground turkey
4 tbs. mango chutney, divided
1/4 tsp. salt
2 cups shredded romaine lettuce

How to Make It:
Preheat grill to medium-high.
Cut baguette into 4 equal lengths. Split each piece horizontally and pull out about half of the soft bread from each side.
Finely chop enough onion rounds to equal 1/3 cup. Combine the chopped onion with turkey, 1 tablespoon chutney and salt in a medium bowl; gently mix with your hands until well combined.

Form into 4 burgers, about 1/2 inch thick and oval-shaped to match the shape of the bread.

Oil the grill rack. Grill the remaining onion rounds until softened and blackened in spots, 3 to 4 minutes per side. Grill the burgers until cooked through and an instant-read thermometer inserted into the center registers 165 F, 4 to 5 minutes per side. Grill the bread, cut-side down, until just beginning to char on the edges, about 2 minutes.

To assemble sandwiches, spread the remaining mango chutney on the bottom pieces of baguette. Top with a turkey burger, grilled onion and lettuce. Cover with the remaining bread.

Snack:

Homemade Trail Mix.

The trail mix you buy in stores is often nothing more than a sugary candy mix, but by making your own custom mix with roasted nuts and unsweetened dried fruits you'll have an energy packed snack that keeps you going!

Healthy Eating Meal Plan – Day 4

Breakfast:
Green Smoothie.
Green smoothies are an awesome way to set the day for a day full of healthy eating. Add a handful of greens, a frozen banana, a few blueberries, and enough milk/milk alternative to reach your preferred consistency to the blender to create a dynamic green smoothie.

Lunch:
Bento Box.
Bento boxes are a hot trend among kids' lunchboxes, but you can use the trend to make a healthy lunch full of variety for yourself. Pack a small portion of several choices like roasted nuts, steamed veggies, boiled eggs, cheese, and fruit in separate compartments for a fun and healthy lunch.

Dinner:
Steak Kabobs.
Think steak is off limits in a healthy diet? Think again! Lean cuts of beef can provide much needed iron and vitamins.

What You'll Need:
1 1/2 pounds beef sirloin steak, cut 1 inch thick, and/or skinless, boneless chicken breasts and/or thighs
1/2 cup barbecue sauce
1/4 cup water
2 - 4 garlic, minced
2 tbs. dried minced onion
2 tbs. sugar
2 tbs. steak sauce
2 tbs. vinegar
2 tbs. Worcestershire sauce
2 tbs. cooking oil
1/2 tsp. salt
2 medium onions, each cut into 8 wedges
10 - 12 medium fresh button mushrooms, stems removed

1 medium zucchini, halved and sliced 1/2 inch thick
1 large red or green sweet pepper, cut into 1-inch pieces

How to Make It:
Cut steak into 1-inch cubes. Or, cut chicken into 1-inch pieces.
Put steak and/or chicken in a plastic bag set in a shallow dish.
For Marinade:
In a saucepan, mix the barbecue sauce, water, garlic, dried onion, sugar, steak sauce, vinegar, Worcestershire, oil, and salt. Bring to just boiling. Cool. Pour over steak or chicken; seal bag. Marinate in refrigerator for 6 to 8 hours or overnight.
In a saucepan, cook onions, covered, in small amount of boiling water for 3 minutes. Add mushrooms; cook for 1 minute more. Drain. Thread vegetables onto five 6-inch metal skewers with zucchini and sweet pepper pieces.
Drain meat, reserving marinade; thread meat onto five 6-inch metal skewers. Cook on rack of uncovered grill over medium heat for 12 to 14 minutes or till done, turning halfway through. In saucepan, heat marinade until bubbly.
Grill vegetables over medium heat for 5 to 10 minutes, turning occasionally; brush with heated marinade.
Serve immediately with warm marinade.

Snack:
Fruit Dippers.
Slice up your favorite fruits and dip them fondue style in plain yogurt swirled with a teaspoon of honey and cinnamon to taste for a fun and easy snack full of antioxidants!

Healthy Eating Meal Plan – Day 5

Breakfast:
Savory Breakfast Bowl.
Use sautéed greens of your choice as the base of your breakfast bowl, top with lean chicken sausage, and diced sweet potato. Somewhat unconventional for breakfast, but this filling, protein packed breakfast will keep you going without weighing you down.

Lunch:
Tuna Stuffed Avocado.
Pit an avocado and fill with canned wild caught tuna. Sprinkle with salt and pepper and a squeeze of lemon juice. Enjoy with an apple on the side.

Dinner:
Loaded Greek Salad.
This flavorful Greek salad has it all. Top with grilled chicken for added protein.

What You'll Need:
2 cups Romaine lettuce
1/4 cup chopped red onions
1/4 cup chopped cucumbers
2 ounces feta cheese
8 olives
2 tbs. red wine vinegar
1 tsp. oregano

How to Make It:
Combine all ingredients in a bowl.
Add vinegar and oregano and toss salad.

Snack:
Dark Chocolate Delight.

Choose a dark chocolate of at least 80 percent cacao content and enjoy about 2 ounces alongside orange wedges for a combo that's delightful!

Healthy Eating Meal Plan – Day 6

Breakfast:
Power Parfait.
Layer plain Greek yogurt with berries and toasted oats for a breakfast that tastes like a dessert, but fuels you up!

Lunch:
Greek Salad Pita.
Use leftovers from your salad last night to fill half a whole grain tortilla for an easy and tasty lunch.

Dinner:
Cauliflower Stir Fry.
Using riced cauliflower instead of rice is a perfect way to cut carbs and calories and sneak in an extra serving of veggies!

What You'll Need:
1 medium head (about 24 oz) cauliflower, rinsed
1 tbs. sesame oil
2 egg whites
1 large egg
pinch of salt
cooking spray
1/2 small onion, diced fine
1/2 cup frozen peas and carrots
2 garlic cloves, minced
5 scallions, diced, whites and greens separated
3 tbs. soy sauce

How to Make It:
Remove the core and let the cauliflower dry completely. Coarsely chop into florets, then place half of the cauliflower in a food processor and pulse until the cauliflower is small and has the texture of rice or couscous – don't over process or it will get mushy. Set aside and repeat with the remaining cauliflower.

Snack:

Better Banana Split.

Split a banana in half length wise and spread with your favorite nut butter, unsweetened coconut flakes, and dark chocolate chips. Tastes decadent, but loaded with nutrition!

Healthy Eating Meal Plan – Day 7

Breakfast:
Pumpkin oatmeal.
Pumpkin is loaded with vitamins and fiber, but all you'll think about with this oatmeal is how yummy it is!

What You'll Need:
1 (14-ounce) can pumpkin puree (the unseasoned kind)
2 cups water
2 cups unsweetened almond milk, or water
2 tbs. raisins (golden or regular)
1/4 tsp. kosher salt
3/4 tsp. pumpkin pie spice OR 1/2 tsp. cinnamon plus 1/4 tsp. ground
cardamom plus 1/4 tsp. ground cloves
2 cups quick cooking oatmeal (not the instant kind)
1/4 cup pepitas (pumpkin seeds)
Honey or maple sugar, for serving
Heavy cream, for serving

How to Make It:
In large saucepan over high heat, combine the pumpkin puree, water, milk, raisins, salt, and pumpkin pie spice (alternative spices). Bring to a boil.
Add the oatmeal. Turn the heat down and cook according to your oatmeal instructions; mine usually takes about 15 minutes. Stir often.
Meanwhile, in a small cast iron skillet over medium heat, toast the pepitas until they're fragrant and a gentle golden brown, about 10 minutes.
Once the oatmeal is cooked (each grain should be tender), serve with honey or maple sugar on the side, pepitas to sprinkle on top, and cream if people like it more like porridge.

Lunch:
Quick Quesadilla.

Fill a whole grain or gluten free tortilla with loads of spinach, slices of avocado, and a sprinkle of cheese. Pan fry in coconut oil for a crispy finish or microwave if you're pressed for time.

Dinner:

Quinoa Bake.
Looking for a meatless meal that still provides plenty of protein?

What You'll Need:
3-3/4 cup chicken broth, divided
1-1/2 cups dry quinoa, rinsed very well under cold running water
2 cups small broccoli florets
4 tbs. butter, divided
8 oz sliced mushrooms
1 shallot or 1/4 small onion, chopped
salt and pepper
3 cloves garlic, minced
2 tbs. gluten-free flour
1 cup milk
3 oz freshly shredded Monterey Jack cheese
3 oz freshly shredded sharp cheddar cheese

How to Make It:
Preheat oven to 350 F. Spray an 8×8 baking dish with nonstick spray then place on top of a baking sheet and set aside.
Bring 2-3/4 cups chicken broth to a boil in a medium-sized saucepan then add quinoa, place a lid on top, turn heat down to medium, and then simmer until nearly all the liquid has been absorbed and quinoa is tender, 20 minutes. Add broccoli then place lid back on top, remove from heat, and let steam for 10 minutes.
Meanwhile, melt 2 Tablespoons butter in a large skillet over medium-high heat. Add mushrooms and shallots, season with salt and pepper, then saute until mushrooms are golden brown. Add garlic then saute for one more minute.
Add remaining 2 Tablespoons butter then sprinkle in flour when melted and saute for one minute. Slowly stream in remaining 1

cup chicken broth and milk while whisking to avoid lumps. Season generously with salt and pepper then bring mixture to a bubble while stirring constantly. Turn heat down to medium then simmer until thick and bubbly, 5 minutes.

Remove from heat then stir in the broccoli and quinoa, and half the cheese, then scoop mixture into prepared baking dish. Sprinkle remaining cheese on top then bake for 15-20 minutes, or until cheese is golden brown and bubbly.

Snack:
Granola Protein Bites.
Try these yummy bites as a snack or a protein packed dessert. Make a large batch to have these around all week!

What You'll Need:
1 cup oats
2/3 cup toasted shredded coconut
1/2 cup peanut butter
1/2 cup mini chocolate chips
1/3 cup honey
1 tbs. chia seeds
1 tsp. vanilla

How to Make It:
Combine all ingredients in a large bowl.
Roll and compress the mixture into 1 inch rounds and place on parchment paper
Refrigerate a few minutes until firm and then transfer to an air tight container.
Refrigerate and enjoy for up to one week.

Healthy Eating Meal Plan – Day 8

Breakfast:
Banana "Pancake."
Imagine a pancake that doesn't leave you feeling sluggish, but instead nourishes you for your morning.

What You'll Need:
1 mashed, super ripe banana
2 eggs
Coconut oil for the pan
Optional: a bit of pumpkin pie spice, 2 tbs. of ground flaxseed, a bit of vanilla, & a dash of cinnamon, all-natural maple syrup + berries

How to Make It:
Smash your banana with a fork. In another bowl whisk eggs. Mix eggs & banana together. Put the coconut oil in the pan. Add a silver dollar-sized amount to the pan. Let the cake set for thirty seconds and flip it! Enjoy with berries and a bit of syrup.

Lunch:
Salad in a Jar.
Layer spinach leaves, chopped boiled egg, nuts, diced tomato, and grilled chicken in a jar for a salad that's perfectly portable and perfectly tasty. Add olive oil and vinegar before eating.

Dinner:
Taco Night.
Mexican meals don't have to equal greasy, carb loaded dinners. These lettuce wrapped tacos are a terrific choice for your next taco night!

What You'll Need:
12 ounces boneless skinless chicken breasts, cut into 4-inch-long, 1-inch-thick strips
2 tsp. Mediterranean Spice
1/4 cup Balsamic Vinaigrette

4 romaine lettuce leaves, shredded
1 tbs. thinly sliced red onion
1/4 cup Red-Wine Vinaigrette
1/4 cup Tzatziki
12 butter lettuce leaves
4 Roma tomatoes, chopped
1 1/2 ounces crumbled feta cheese
12 kalamata olives, pitted and chopped
1 tsp. chopped parsley
1/2 tsp. dried basil
1/2 tsp. dried oregano

How to Make It:
Preheat a grill pan over high heat. Season chicken with 1 teaspoon Mediterranean spice and place on grill. Cook, basting with balsamic vinaigrette and turning once, until cooked through, about 2 minutes per side. Season chicken with remaining teaspoon Mediterranean spice and remove from grill; set aside.
Place shredded romaine lettuce and red onions in a medium bowl; drizzle with red-wine vinaigrette and toss to combine. Divide mixture evenly among butter lettuce leaves and drizzle each with 1 teaspoon tzatziki.
Top each taco with 1 piece of chicken and garnish with chopped tomatoes, feta cheese, and olives. Season with parsley, basil, and oregano; serve.

Snack: Fruit Pizza. Spread a thin layer of cream cheese on a toasted whole wheat or low carb tortilla and top with whatever fresh (or frozen) fruits you have around. Sprinkle with cinnamon (optional)

Healthy Eating Meal Plan – Day 9

Breakfast:
Egg Cups.
A complete breakfast in a convenient muffin tin! Follow this recipe, but add in your favorite chopped veggies.

What You'll Need:
Eggs
Ham or Turkey (I used smoked turkey)
(Optional) Scallions or what ever you like with your eggs!

How to Make It:
Preheat your oven to 400 F.
Grease up your Muffin/Cupcake Pan. You can either spray it down with some cooking spray, or you can do what I did which was smear some Coconut Oil all over it.
Fit 1 or 2 slices of ham in to each muffin cup. I used two because my ham was sliced real thin.
(Optional) Depending on if you want your eggs all scrambled or not, you can crack an egg in to a separate cup and beat it before dumping it in to the ham cups. If you do decide on doing this, you can also mix in your other ingredients (think chopped mushrooms/scallions/spinach).
If you like your eggs whole, go ahead and crack that egg in to the cup!
(Optional) Throw a few pieces of your chopped up scallions on top for garnish!
Pop that muffin pan in to the oven which you previously preheated 400 F and bake for 15 minutes or however well you like your eggs.

Lunch:
Burrito Bowl.
Copy this popular restaurant menu item by layering beans, lettuce, chopped tomatoes, sliced chicken, salsa and avocado to create a burrito bowl at your own house. Go sparingly on the

cheese and brown rice, or omit them entirely if calories are a concern.

Dinner:
Stuffed Bell Peppers.
Fill this super food with everything you need for dinner and you'll have an easy to make dinner loaded with nutrients in no time.

What You'll Need:
4 large green bell peppers
1 1/2 tsp. canola oil
1 medium onion, chopped
1 clove garlic, minced
1 pound ground turkey
1 1/2 cups cooked rice
1 8-ounce can tomato sauce, (1 cup), divided
1 tbs. chopped fresh parsley
1 tsp. salt, (optional)
1/4 tsp. freshly ground pepper

How to Make It:
Preheat oven to 350 F.
Cut out stem ends of bell peppers and discard. Scoop out seeds. Bring 8 cups water to a boil in a large pot and blanch the peppers until tender-crisp, about 1 minute. Drain and cool under cold running water. Set aside.
Heat oil in a large nonstick skillet over medium heat. Add onion and garlic and cook, stirring occasionally, until softened, about 3 minutes. Add turkey and cook, crumbling with a wooden spoon, just until it loses its pink color, about 2 minutes. Drain the fat. Transfer the turkey mixture to a medium bowl and mix in rice, 1/2 cup tomato sauce, parsley, salt (if using) and pepper. Stuff the peppers with the mixture and place them in a 2-quart casserole dish. Spoon the remaining 1/2 cup tomato sauce over the peppers. Cover and bake until the peppers are tender and the filling is heated through, 30 to 35 minutes.

Snack:
Hummus and Raw Veggies.
Protein, healthy fat, fiber, antioxidants...this snack has it all.
Make your own hummus or use store bought, but either way
make sure you insisting on quality ingredients.

Healthy Eating Meal Plan – Day 10

Breakfast:
'Better than Cereal' Cereal.
Walk the cereal aisle and you'll find many blood sugar spiking, energy draining options full of artificial ingredients and sugar. Make your own "cereal" by pouring your favorite milk/milk alternative over unsweetened coconut flakes, chopped fruit, hemp hearts, and a spoonful of your favorite nut butter for a satisfying cereal sure to beat any boxed cereal.

Lunch:
New and Improved Chicken Salad.
Use your favorite chicken salad recipe, but cut out the mayo and replace it with avocado instead. Fill celery stalks with the chicken salad for a crunch. Grapes make a terrific side!

Dinner:
Sweet Potato Crusted Spinach Quiche.
Take away the unhealthy crust found on most quiches and you actually have a healthy option filled with veggies and proteins. These sweet potatoes add fiber, vitamins and loads of flavor. Best of all, it's a complete meal in one dish! Strawberries are a perfect dessert to end your meal!

What You'll Need:
6 small sweet potatoes
A bunch of spinach
Half of a small onion
1 clove of garlic
4 eggs
1 cup of grated mozzarella (try to use it fresh, it's always better!)
Spring herbs of your choice (we recommend dill, because it is marvelous in a quiche!)
1/4 cup of goat cheese
1/4 cup of asiago cheese
Salt & Pepper to taste

How to Make It:

Peel the sweet potatoes and slice them thinly.

Lay the slices in the bottom of a pie dish, in a crust-like fashion.

Spray with a little bit of extra virgin olive oil and bake at 400 F for 15 minutes.

In a little bit of oil, sauté the onion and garlic until golden brown. Then, add in the spinach and sauté for 4 minutes.

Drain it over the sink and get rid of the excess liquid.

In a bowl, blend eggs and mozzarella.

Add, in the bowl, the herbs and goat cheese. Then, add the spinach-onion-garlic mixture to the bowl.

Pour over the potato crust and sprinkle the asiago cheese on top.

Bake at 375 F for 40 minutes, or until the quiche is firm and the cheese browned.

Snack:

Homemade Protein Bar.

Many protein bars on the market are filled with artificial preservatives that aren't good for anyone! Make your own by combining equal parts walnuts and unsweetened dried fruits. If you don't have the time to make your own protein bars, look for an option with only nuts and fruit and you'll be all set!

Healthy Eating Meal Plan – Day 11

Breakfast:
Leftover Quiche.
Last night's sweet potato quiche reheats beautifully for a quick breakfast you'll look forward to all night (hint: save the recipe from dinner to make for an impressive brunch go-to!)

Lunch:
Cucumber Stackers.
Stack slices of cucumbers with lean deli meat, chicken salad, or tuna for a sandwich with a crunch. Use mustard and hummus for condiments. Have about 1/4 cup of almonds for a side.

Dinner:
Black Bean Soup.
Choose your favorite of these five super food soup recipes for a healing, healthy dinner. Use whole grain bread toasted in place of croutons.

What You'll Need:
1 (15-oz) can black beans, drained and rinsed
1 tbs. extra-virgin olive oil
1 cup onion, small diced
2 tbs. fresh garlic, minced
1/2 tsp. dried oregano
1/2 tsp. paprika
1/4 tsp. cumin
2 cups water and 1 tbs. natural vegetable base (or 2 cups vegetable stock)
1/3 cup poblano pepper, charred, peeled, seeded and chopped (approximately 1
poblano pepper)
2 tbs. tomato paste

How to Make It:
In cook pot on medium heat, add oil and sauté onion until transparent.

Add garlic and sauté two minutes. Add remaining ingredients. Bring to a simmer, turn off heat, then remove from stove and purée with vertical immersion blender until puréed. Serve or allow to cool, and then cover, label, date and refrigerate.

Snack:
Flourless Muffin.
Part treat, part snack, all healthy. Everyone is sure to love these flourless muffins

What You'll Need:
1/2 cup unsweetened apple sauce
1/2 cup peanut butter
1 egg
1/4 tsp. baking soda
3 tbs. honey
1 tbs. pure vanilla extract
1/4 tsp. salt
1 tsp. cinnamon
1/2 tsp. ground ginger
1/8 tsp. ground cloves
3/4-1 cup diced apple (from about 1 medium apple)

How to Make It:
Preheat your oven to 400 F. Grease a mini muffin pan and set aside. In a blender, blend all ingredients except the diced apple very well. Stir in the apple (don't blend it). Fill each muffin cup almost to the top. Bake for 10 minutes. Allow to cool completely before removing from the tray (they will stick if you don't let them cool first).

Healthy Eating Meal Plan – Day 12

Breakfast:
Almond Flour Muffin.
The almond flour used in these muffins cuts the carbs and makes them far more filling than ordinary muffins.

What You'll Need:
4 ounces blanched almond flour (not almond meal) (about 1 cup)
4 ounces eggs (about 2 large eggs)
1 ounce honey (around 1 tbs.)
1/4 tsp. baking soda
1/2 tsp. apple cider vinegar

How to Make It:
In a medium bowl, combine almond flour and baking soda.
In a large bowl combine eggs, honey and vinegar.
Stir dry ingredients into wet, mixing until combined.
Scoop about 1/4 cup of batter at a time into a paper lined muffin pan.
Bake at 350 F for 15 minutes, until slightly browned around the edges.
Cool in the pan for 1/2 hour.
Serve with butter and jam.

Lunch:
Soup 'To Go'.
Pack a thermos full of last night's soup for today's lunch! As the flavors blend, it may just be better than the night before!

Dinner:
Portabella Pizzas.
Pizza night doesn't have to derail your healthy eating goals any longer!

What You'll Need:

6 portobello mushroom caps, washed and dried with stems removed
1/2 cup tomato sauce (you can use your favorite jarred pasta sauce)
1 tbs. fresh garlic, minced
1/4 cup sliced black olives
1/4 cup sliced mini sweet peppers
1/4 cup minced red onion
Cherry tomatoes, sliced (use what you feel is a desirable amount for each pizza)
Fresh mozzarella cheese, sliced (package sizes vary from 5-8 ounces, just use what you feel is necessary for each pizza)
Fresh basil for garnish (optional)
1 tbs. of Italian seasonings, divided

How to Make It:
Preheat the oven to 375 F and line a baking sheet with parchment paper. Place the mushroom, cap side up, on a baking sheet and bake for 5 minutes.
Remove the mushrooms from the oven and spoon the tomato sauce into the center of each mushroom cap. Top with cheese, sliced tomatoes, olives, sliced peppers, minced red onion and garlic. Bake for an additional 20 minutes, or until cheese is melted and golden.
Garnish each pizza with fresh basil and Italian seasonings and serve immediately.

Snack:
Kale Chips and Salsa.
Kale chips are all the rage for good reason. They are a super food combined with all the goodness of chips! Add even more flavor and antioxidants by dipping them in salsa!

Healthy Eating Meal Plan – Day 13

Breakfast:
Very Berry Smoothie.
Green smoothies get to be the star of the smoothie world, but this beet and berry smoothie will give them some stiff competition (also perfect for anyone who is apprehensive of the green smoothie!)

What You'll Need:
1 medium beet, steamed, roasted, or raw (if you don't have a high speed blender,
use steamed or roasted)
1 cup fresh or frozen mixed berries
1/2 cup fresh orange, sectioned
3/4 cup homemade almond milk or 3/4 cup commercial almond milk and 1 tbs. hempseed

How to Make It:
Blend all ingredients together, and serve with orange sections for color!

Lunch:
Deli Meat Pizza.
Pizza becomes even easier when you top a slice of nitrate-free deli meat with marinara, veggies, and cheese. Just microwave to cook. Enjoy extra veggies to complete your meal.

Dinner:
Fish in Parchment.
Use this recipe for a quick and healthy way to cook the fish of your choice and serve with a side of quinoa and roasted Brussels sprouts.

What You'll Need:
1 (6-ounce) firm-fleshed white-fish fillet, such as halibut, cod, or haddock (the fillet should be between 3/4 and 1 1/4 inches thick)

1 tbs. extra-virgin olive oil
Salt
Freshly ground black pepper
1 bay leaf, cut in half (optional)
Fresh herbs, such as chives, parsley, tarragon, or chervil (optional)
1 tbs. unsalted butter
3 thin lemon slices
1 tbs. dry white wine or water

How to Make It:
Heat the oven to 400 F and arrange a rack in the middle.
Draw out a large piece of parchment paper (about 17 by 11 inches) and, with one of the longer edges closest you, fold it in half from left to right. Using scissors, cut out a large heart shape.
Place the fish in the center of one half of the parchment heart. (The heart should be large enough that there is at least a 1-1/2-inch border around the fillet.) Set the parchment heart on a baking sheet. Drizzle the fish with half of the olive oil, rub the oil all over the fillet, and season with salt and pepper.
Lay half of the bay leaf and a few sprigs of herbs (if using) on top of the fish. Break the butter into little pieces and arrange them on top of the herbs.
Place the lemon slices over everything and drizzle with the remaining oil.
Fold the parchment heart over to cover the fish. (The edges of the heart should line up.) Starting at the rounded end, crimp the edges together, folding them over themselves and leaving the last two inches at the pointed end unfolded. Slightly tilt the package up and pour in the wine or water. Finish crimping the edges, then twist the pointed end around once and fold the "tail" under.
Place the baking sheet in the oven and bake 10 minutes for a 3/4-inch-thick fillet or 12 minutes for a 1- to 1-1/4-inch-thick fillet.
Remove the baking sheet from the oven and transfer the parchment package to a dinner plate. Serve immediately, cutting into the parchment tableside using scissors or a knife.

Snack:
Brown Rice Cake, Peanut Butter, and Honey.
All of these ingredients are easy to keep on hand at home or in the office at any time. Sprinkle with cinnamon for extra flavor and antioxidants!

Healthy Eating Meal Plan – Day 14

Breakfast:
Sweet Breakfast Bowl.
Consider this bowl the counterpart to the savory breakfast bowl you had earlier in the plan. Top your favorite smoothie with nuts, fruit, and hemp hearts and/or chia seeds.

Lunch:
Loaded Sweet Potato.
Microwave or bake a small sweet potato and top with black beans, broccoli, sliced chicken, and olive oil for a lunch that will be the envy of everyone around you.

Dinner:
Shrimp and Zoodles.
You'll never missed the refined carbs when you replace zoodles with noodles!

What You'll Need:
1 1/2 tsp. olive oil
pinch crushed red pepper flakes
4 oz peeled and deveined shrimp
2 cloves garlic, sliced thin and devided
1 medium zucchini, spiralized
pinch salt and fresh black pepper
1/4 lemon
1/4 cup halved grape tomatoes

How to Make It:
Heat a medium nonstick skillet over medium-high heat. Add 1 teaspoon of the oil and crush red pepper flakes, add the shrimp and season with pinch salt and pepper; cook 2 to 3 minutes. Add half of the garlic and continue cooking 1 more minute, or until the shrimp is cooked through and opaque. Set aside on a dish.

Snack:
Black bean brownies.

If you are looking for a treat that won't derail your healthy goals, this is for you.

What You'll Need:
1 1/2 cups black beans (1 15-oz can, drained and rinsed very well) (250g after draining)
2 tbs. cocoa powder (10g)
1/2 cup quick oats (40g)
1/4 tsp. salt
1/3 cup pure maple syrup or agave (or honey, but not for strict vegans.) (75g)
pinch uncut stevia OR 2 tbs. sugar (or omit and increase maple syrup to 1/2 cup)
1/4 cup coconut or vegetable oil (40g)
2 tsp. pure vanilla extract
1/2 tsp. baking powder
1/2 cup to 2/3 cup chocolate chips (115-140g)

How to Make It:
Preheat oven to 350 F. Combine all ingredients except chips in a good food processor, and blend until completely smooth. Really blend well. (A blender can work if you absolutely must, but the texture—and even the taste—will be much better in a food processor.) Stir in the chips, then pour into a greased 8×8 pan. Optional: sprinkle extra chocolate chips over the top. Cook the black bean brownies 15-18 minutes, then let cool at least 10 minutes before trying to cut. If they still look a bit undercooked, you can place them in the fridge overnight and they will magically firm up!

Now that your 14 days are over, there's a still little to add. Fitness is not just achieved by checking up on the meals you take alone, it also entail many weeks of training- it's about the physiological and psychological balance of the body. You cannot be applauded with a fabulous body just by going through this pocket guide alone without putting some work in to it.

What's stopping you?
Whatever it is that's stopping you from getting more active and staying fit, it might not be as much of a barrier as you think. You might be considering certain things as reasons why you might avoid exercise; time shouldn't a barrier- achieving about 140-150 minutes of physical activity a week is easier than you think, just give it a try today! You definitely have the willpower; a lot of people give up on their exercise regime soon after starting it. One of the way to stay fit and lose excess fat is to stay on track, and work towards a target that suits you.

Let's take you through exercise motivation- the next step to start losing weight right now

Did you know? The muscles and flesh you didn't even know you had are giving you grief and it may feel like a bit of an uphill struggle- this is not just your body. One of the biggest barriers to getting on with exercises routine is your mind. We're creatures of habit, and if you have not done much for a while, looking for the motivation to get up and start can be a real mental battle. But don't get discouraged, you'd only go through the beginner's plan barrier and after a week or two; it would be a distant memory. If at any point you feel your enthusiasm relapsing at any point, here are top ten tips to boost your morale and get you on the run!

Be realistic: always remind yourself that you have to become active and fit, since that's the only way to become healthier and lose weight. It's a crucial component of your 14- day journey.

Schedule it: plan your exercise alongside preparation for your meals, probably at the start of the week and put it in your diary. Planning in advance when, how, and where you will carry out your exercising activity will increase your chances of making physical activity a normal part of your lifestyle. You might even go around with simple approaches like laying out your running kit or packing your gym bag at night before can help.

Pat yourself at the back: don't forget you've gone this far because you have a focus, always look back at your weekly food and activity plan and remind yourself how much you've already achieved.

Don't keep the word! Spread it: make sure to share your plans and achievements with other people planning to kick start, with that you'll feel obliged to keep going!

Set goals: they don't need to be big achievements; for instance, try to take a walk a little more bit more each day, take the stairs instead of the lift or walk half or part of the way to work. Keeping a written record of these mini goals will help you to view your progress over time.

At work? There are still some things to put in to consideration.

Since you'll spend about third of your day at work, so it will make sense to give you what you should eat during work hours. Below are 10 tips to make workplace eating healthier for you?

Take breakfast: as explained earlier, this should be your mantra. A healthier breakfast will keep you going for the day and prevent you from becoming hungry before lunch time. Even if you're not feeling the urge to eat in the morning before leaving for work, have breakfast at work.

Bring your own: the recipes that have been listed earlier should be followed; home- made food is often lower in calories and fat, and even cheaper than food bought on the street, or in a cafeteria. If you do not like sandwiches, you could cook extra in the evenings and take the leftovers to work, saving you money and excess fat.

Drink water: taking water regularly will help keep hunger pangs on check. At least, take about drink to eight glasses; around 1.2 liters of fluid every day.

Plan your snacks: healthier snack alone should be kept within reach; fruits like carrot sticks and reduced fat- hummus dip shouldn't be far from you.

Go 'low mayo': try only lower fat mayonnaise, since it contains about 80% fat, and just a few dollops can turn a healthier meal in to an unhealthy one.

Conclusion

Thank You again for downloading this book.
I hope this book was able to help You to flatten your belly.

Finally, if You enjoyed this book, then I'd like to ask You for a favor, would You be kind enough to leave a review for this book on Amazon? It'd be greatly appreciated!

Thank You and good luck!

www.ingramcontent.com/pod-product-compliance
Lightning Source LLC
Chambersburg PA
CBHW050848290526
45792CB00002B/565